Myocardial Protection- A Brief Overview

Myocardial Protection

A Brief Overview

FAHEEM IQBAL

NOTION PRESS

Myocardial Protection- A Brief Overview

NOTION PRESS

India. Singapore. Malaysia.

Myocardial Protection- A Brief Overview

Dedicated to my family, teachers and friends.

Myocardial Protection- A Brief Overview

Myocardial Protection

Faheem Iqbal

Myocardial Protection- A Brief Overview

CONTENTS

Myocardial Protection- A Brief Overview

1. Introduction

- **Myocardial Protection involves a set of techniques that are employed during the cardiac surgery to augment the heart's ability to withstand the injury caused by *ischemia* and *reperfusion*.**

- **The *still* and *bloodless* operating conditions required for cardiac surgery are detrimental to the metabolic demands of the heart, therefore, to prevent further injury, a comprehensive myocardial protection strategy, involving the conduct of operation before, during and after the period of ischemia is required.**

- **This booklet is a brief discussion on the myocardial protection, involving its history and methods, with special reference to cardioplegia.**

2. History

- **The earliest cardiac procedures utilised myocardial cooling accompanied by systemic hypothermia to facilitate the conduct of surgery, and not as a means of myocardial protection.**

- **In 1955, <u>Melrose</u> introduced the concept of reversible hyperkalemic cardiac arrest in order to improve surgical exposure; it, however caused myocardial quiescence and was hence abandoned.**

- In 1956, <u>Lillehei</u> proposed the use of retrograde coronary perfusion as a method of myocardial protection.

- In 1961, <u>Hufnagel</u> etal. introduced topical myocardial cooling by the use of ice cold saline and slush.

- In 1964, <u>Bretschneider</u> introduced calcium free, procaine containing cardioplegia solution.

- In 1967, <u>Taber</u> etal. were the first to associate myocardial injury with poor myocardial protection.

- In 1973, <u>Gay</u> & <u>Ebert</u> reintroduced hyperkalemic cardioplegia, but with lower potassium concentrations as compared to Melrose and showed that it could arrest the heart for about 60 ms, without causing any cellular damage.

- In 1975, <u>Hearse</u> etal. developed St. Thomas solution.

- In 1978, <u>Follette</u> etal. popularised the use of blood in cardioplegia.

- In 1984, <u>Akins</u> introduced fibrillatory arrest as an alternative to chemical cardioplegia.

- In 1986, <u>Murry</u> introduced ischemic preconditioning.

- 1991, <u>Lichtenstein</u> introduced warm blood cardioplegia.

- In 1995, <u>Pedro</u> etal. introduced del Nido cardioplegia solution at Boston children's hospital.

3. Methods of Myocardial Protection

- **Various methods have been used to protect the myocardium during the cardiac surgery, as discussed follows.**

1. Cardioplegia

- **It plays a very important role to alter or inhibit the ischemic injury by utilising diastolic asystole and hypothermia and avoids reperfusion injury by utilising various pharmacological agents like mannitol, magnesium, adenosine, etc.**

2. Ischemic Preconditioning

- **Brief periods of nonlethal ischemia and reperfusion are utilised to enable the heart to tolerate a subsequent longer period of ischemia (and reperfusion).**

- **It has been shown to reduce troponin leakage, myocardial dysfunction and arrhythmias in procedures employing cardioplegic attest.**

3. Ischemic Postconditioning

- **It involves the administration of medications at the time of initial reperfusion after clamp removal to minimise ischemic-reperfusion injury;**

eg. adenosine (1.5mg/kg) and mannitol (1-2ml/kg) may be administered.

4. Fibrillatory Arrest:-

- Intermittent aortic clamping combined with fibrillatory arrest and systemic hypothermia (30-32°C) is an established myocardial protection technique in some surgeries especially CABG.

- Induction of VF reduces cardiac motion, thereby facilitating suturing of distal graft anastomosis in 10-15 ms ischemic duration, while the proximal anastomosis to the ascending aorta can then be performed with the heart perfused (beating) and the procedure is repeated for another graft.

5. Beating Heart Surgery

- Performing the cardiac surgery on beating heart (on or off pump), whenever feasible, reduces the inflammatory response and hence damage to the myocardium.

6. Venting

- It's used in addition to cardioplegic arrest and prevents distention of the ventricle and ejection of air, reduces myocardial rewarming and provides a bloodless surgical field.

7. Non-Cardioplegic Medications

- These include erythropoietin (limits myocardial injury), N-acetyl cysteine (reduces oxidative stress), deferoxemine (reduces hydroxyl radical formation), statins (possess antioxidative and anti-inflammatory properties).

4. Cardiolegia

The chemically induced, deliberate and temporary cessation of the heart's activity during the cardiac surgery is known as the cardioplegia and the solution used for this purpose is known as the cardioplegia solution.

The agent commonly used to arrest the heart is potassium, hence the cardioplegia solutions are usually hyperkalemic.

It was introduced by Melrose in 1955.

The term cardioplegia was coined by CR Lam in 1957.

This chapter discusses the various types and methods of cardioplegia and also provides a brief overview of its significance.

4.1 Types of cardioplegia

Based on their formulations, cardioplegia solutions can be called intracellular or extracellular.

Intracellular solutions use potassium as the arresting agent and usually contain no sodium or calcium, which generates a large osmolar space, which is available for other potentially protective components, e.g., mannitol, dextrose, histidine, glucose, etc.

Extracellular solutions contain calcium and sodium, the primary determinants of transcellular calcium exchange and only a moderate amount of potassium and magnesium.

Cardioplegia solutions are also classified as crystalloid and blood solutions.

Crystalloid solutions contain four parts of crystalloid and one part of blood. An important example is that of del Nido cardioplegia, which contains potassium, magnesium, mannitol, sodium bicarbonate and lidocaine in one litre of the plasmalyte A.

Blood cardioplegia contains four parts of blood and one part of crystalloid. An important example is that of Sanguine St. Thomas cardioplegia, which contains 32 mmols of potassium, 32 mmols of magnesium, calcium, sodium bicarbonate, procaine and adenosine in one litre of Ringer's lactate.

4.2 Methods of Cardioplegia Delivery

There are basically two methods to deliver cardioplegia (antegrade and retrograde), each with their own merits and demirits.

Antegrade cardioplegia involves the placement of a short needle tip antegrade cannula, with or without vent port, into the aortic root between the aortic valve and the aortic cross clamp; both prevent flow in either direction, thus forcing the cardioplegia solution in the coronary arteries. Antegrade infusion pressure should be between 80-100 mmHg; high pressures may cause endothelial injury and myocardial edema. Antegrade cardioplegia in case of aortic regurgitation is given directly in coronary ostia using special tip ostial cannula and in case of coronary stenosis, it's supplemented or replaced with retrograde delivery.

Retrograde cardioplegia involves the placement of a balloon-tip catheter into the coronary sinus through the right atrium. The balloon is self-inflating or manually inflatable to prevent the reflux of the cardioplegia solution into the right atrium. Retrograde infusion pressures

shouldn't be exceeded above 50 mmHg to prevent coronary sinus damage.

4.3 Cardioplegia & Ischemia/Reperfusion Injury

Cardioplegia reduces the severity of ischemia by initiating immediate diastolic asystole by causing membrane depolarisation with potassium, thereby avoiding the initial depletion of high energy phosphates.

Activation of K_{ATP} channel limits calcium accumulation and hence calcium mediated injury.

Hypothermic cardioplegia reduces the metabolic rate and thus oxygen demand (from 8ml/min/100g to 0.3ml/min/100g); this small demand is then fully met by intermittent cardioplegia delivery.

Supplementation of cardioplegia solution with metabolic substrates (e.g., glucose, aspartate and glutamate) enhances anaerobic metabolism between the infusions of cardioplegia.

Use of buffers (bicarbonate, THAM, histidine or endogenous) provides either normal or slightly alkaline pH, resulting in better enzyme action and metabolism.

Preventing calcium accumulation using citrate (as CPD), calcium channel blocker or magnesium significantly reduces calcium mediated ischemia/reperfusion injury.

Cardioplegia can prevent myocardial edema by employing hyperosmotic agents like mannitol, glucose, albumin, etc.

Use of allapurinol, adenosine, nitric oxide, SOD/CAT, mannitol prevent neutrophil activation and oxygen radical formation.

5. Summary

Early clinicians didn't focus on the protection of myocardium during the cardiac surgery until poor myocardial protection was shown to cause significant damage to the heart.

Cardioplegia, ischemic preconditioning and postconditioning, fibrillatory arrest, venting, beating heart surgery, off pump surgery and several noncardioplegic medications are used for myocardial protection.

Cardioplegia can be classified into

intracellular and extracellular solutions or crystalloid and blood cardioplegia.

Cardioplegia can be delivered antegradely, retrogradely or through both routes.

Cardioplegia significantly inhibits the ischemic injury by virtue of the diastolic asystole and hypothermia, as well as the reperfusion injury by utilising suitable pharmacological additives.

Myocardial Protection by Faheem Iqbal

Myocardial Protection- A Brief Overview